Wild Orange Essential Oil

Benefits, Properties, Applications, Studies & Recipes

by Ann Sullivan

Published in USA by:

Ann Sullivan
217 N. Seacrest Blvd #9
Boynton Beach
FL 33425

© Copyright 2017

ISBN-13: 978-1545428481
ISBN-10: 1545428484

TABLE OF CONTENTS

Introduction

What are essential oils, and how might they be used for therapeutic purposes?

Essential oils are ultra-potent oils, extracted from plants and flowers that have been utilized in medicine for centuries. Presently, they're most commonly used to supplement pharmaceutical medication, but they can also be an effective alternative to pharmaceuticals in the event that you don't have access to them. Before you dismiss essential oils as a means to support the body's natural defenses against injuries and illness, take a look at the historical evidence of the oils' medicinal competence in practice. Your average age-old medical text will demonstrate that essential oils, herbs, and plenty of other natural ingredients have, for thousands of years, successfully enhanced immune function to meet and defeat any number of ailments and injuries. Though traditional medicine is considered "alternative" now, it was once the gold standard. And, frankly, perhaps it still should be, as these natural age-tested remedies can fortify the body's battlements against everything from simple maladies, like headaches, cuts and bruises, to serious diseases, like cancer.

Essential oils are deemed "essential," because the oils are composed of the "essence" of the plant. The difference between essential oils and other oils – like olive oil or vegetable oil, for instance – is that essential oils have high volatility and reduced fixation, which results in faster evaporation, enabling their popular use in aromatherapy. Even at high temperatures, olive and vegetable oils don't evaporate.

Essential oils are especially necessary when it comes to a major natural or man-made disaster or some potential viral outbreak. In these types of dire situations, you may not have quick access (or any access at all) to your standard pharmaceutical supply; so essential oils, along with other alternative medicines, will be your go-to health aids in the case of social collapse, viral outbreak or devastating natural disaster. When medical access is null and void, alternatives to our modern-day standard are the only chance we have to keep pathogens at bay.

You probably don't realize that you already use essential oils every day. They're in perfumes, shampoos, soaps, ointments...they're even used in furniture polish. Why are they found in so many aromatic products? Well, basically, because essential oils are super concentrated aromatic liquids, so their scent is remarkably strong. Let's put this into perspective: to steam tea, you use a few leaves of peppermint or juniper; to produce a single ounce of essential oil, five whole *pounds* of peppermint or juniper leaves are required. Some sources claim that to produce twelve pounds of essential oil would necessitate an acre of peppermint, juniper, or any other oil you're looking to produce en masse. Unlike vegetable oil, you don't often find concentrated therapeutic-grade essential oils sold by the tubload; instead the oils are often sold in easily carried small, dark bottles, perfect for your GOOD bag (Get Out Of Dodge). Which is exactly what this book is aiming to help you do – get out of dodge with your most vital of essential oils intact, in particular a good supply of wild orange essential oil.

Why wild orange, you ask? Well, in order to get you quickly up to speed on this most essential of oils, below we've provided a condensed synopsis of wild orange, after which we'll outline in greater detail the oil's history, properties, and common therapeutic uses, so that you – the consumer – might have a better understanding of the oil's benefits and applications. We've even provided supportive remedies for pure clove, as well as blended recipes that incorporate the valuable oil. Chapter 3 will further detail past scientific research on wild orange essential oil.

Now, let's get down to it.

Essential Oil 101: the Basics of Wild Orange

Summary: Wild Orange, or Citrus sinensis, has been used for centuries in Chinese medicine. Orange was used primarily for digestive purposes, to stimulate the digestive tract and to reduce spasms. Wild orange does more than that, however; its antibacterial, antifungal, and antidepressant properties make it an exceptional disinfectant, while its sweet scent uplifts, energizes and restores peace. Wild orange can be used to kill pathogens, fungus, and even support the body's defenses against cancer. Cultivated in the Dominican Republic, wild orange is composed of 85-95% limonene, which means it has powerful antioxidant properties, alongside other citrus fruits, like lemon, grapefruit, and tangerine.

Description: Wild Orange oil is commonly extracted through the cold pressed or expressed methods. The citrus rind is most often used. The oil is clear orangish green in color, thin in consistency, and has a medium-to-strong fresh sweet citrus scent.

Uses: Beyond those applications previously mentioned, additional uses for Wild Orange essential oil include strengthening the body's defenses against colds, flu, flatulence, constipation, acid reflux, heartburn, stomachache, indigestion, muscle pain, digestion, gums, mouth, and dull skin. When it comes to the mind, the oil can be mentally uplifting, and so can serve as an anti-depressant. It both calms and re-energizes, restoring peace.

Properties: Antioxidant, antibacterial, antifungal, anti-inflammatory, anticancer, antidepressant, antiseptic, antispasmodic, carminative, digestive, sedative, tonic, choleretic, hypotensive, and stimulant.

Application: Dilute 1:1 with a carrier oil. You can apply topically, inhale directly, diffuse or use as a dietary supplement.

Safety Precautions: Wild Orange oil is generally regarded as safe (GRAS). If pregnant or breastfeeding, always consult with your physician when using essential oils. Wild orange is also photosensitive, so if used topically, avoid direct sunlight for up to 24 hours. If you have sensitive skin, dilute heavily.

Fun facts: Wild Orange is derived from the Sanskrit name for "orange tree."

Though the Chinese have been using the rind of the orange for its medicinal value and the high vitamin C content for centuries, oranges weren't transported from southern China to Europe until 1520 by the Portuguese.

Chapter 1:
Benefits of Wild Orange Essential Oil

Wild orange essential oil offers a number of therapeutic benefits; but you may be wondering what these benefits are. In this chapter, we'll take a closer look at the history of wild orange and its many uses.

Cultivation of Wild Orange

Also known as the "sweet orange," wild orange is of the species, Citrus sinensis, as opposed to Citrus aurantium, which is known as the bitter orange. What's interesting is that all citrus trees come from this same genus, Citrus. This means that they are almost entirely interfertile, resulting in a number of specie hybrids. Oranges, grapefruits, lemons, limes – all these fruits come from the same superspecies. Oranges, in fact, have been cultivated for millennia and are believed to be hybrids of mandarins and pomelos (Citrus reticulate and Citrus maxima, respectively). Today, they are the most cultivated fruit the world over, accounting for around 70% of international citrus production, with a large portion of that coming from Florida, California, and Brazil.

Orange trees love water and sunshine and thrive in tropical and subtropical locations, with moderate climates between 60-84°F. The orange tree is a flowering evergreen, generally growing to a height of 30-33 feet. It is not often commercially propagated with seeds, as the seeds are quite often infertile. Instead, the leafy buds of mature trees are grafted into the bark of a seedling rootstock. The tree produces oval leaves around 2.6-3.9 inches long, and oranges that vary in size. Almost all oranges have ten segments and around six seeds inside, along with "pith," the porous white tissue around the rind. The fruit is green when unripe and orange (of course) when ripe.

The Citrus sinensis species is further divided into four classes: the common orange, navel orange, acidless orange, and blood orange.

Common oranges make up about two-thirds of all production, with most of the supply being used for juice. The Valencia orange is an example of this common class. The Valencia ripens in the late-season and, thereby, takes the place of navel oranges when they are out of season.

Navel oranges have a long growing season and wide distribution, making them a very popular orange. Navel oranges are termed thus, because they grow a second fruit at the axis which projects somewhat, similarly to a human navel. Most of the navel orange production is intended for human consumption, because this class of oranges is seedless, produces less juice, and tastes slightly more bitter, making navels less viable for juice making. This class of oranges is believed to have originated from a single mutation in an orange tree at a Brazilian monastery sometime around 1810 and introduced into Florida around 1835. Because the oranges do not produce seeds, they are propagated through cutting and grafting and, thereby, can be considered direct clones of the original fruit's genetic makeup.

Acidless oranges have – as the name would suggest – extremely low levels of acid, which means they aren't suitable for juice processing, as the acid often serves to protect against spoilage. The fruit is cultivated in the early part of the season and is mainly produced for human consumption. They are almost entirely locally consumed, as the spoilage potential means that international export isn't viable.

Though blood oranges were originally a natural mutation of the sinensis species, many of the fruits today are hybrids. Cultivated in Sicily around the 15th century, blood oranges are dark red in color, due to the anthocyanin in their rinds. The blood orange is often deemed the most distinctly flavorful orange and is used in making juice and marmalade. Today blood oranges are mainly cultivated in Italy and Spain.

A History of Wild Orange

The word "orange" is derived from the Sanskrit for "orange tree," which found its way into Late Middle English via Old French. The color was actually named after the fruit sometime around the 16th century.

History indicates that the orange originated in the wild either in northeastern India, southern China, or southeastern Asia. The fruit was first cultivated in China around 2500 BC. They were only introduced to Europe in the 11th century by the crusaders, specifically the bitter orange to Italy. Southern Italy began to cultivate the bitter orange, using it primarily for medical purposes. The sweet orange didn't arrive until around the early 16th century, when the fruit was brought into the Mediterranean by Portuguese and Italian merchants. Thereafter, it was designated a luxury and cultivated for consumption by the upper class. It only came into widespread public consciousness in Europe around the mid 16th century.

The Spanish brought the sweet orange to Americas. It is believed that Christopher Columbus may have transported the fruit to Hispaniola on his second voyage there. The expeditions that followed around the mid 16th century delivered sweet oranges to Mexico, South America and Florida. Missionaries were also largely responsible for the fruits' spread through America; Spanish missionaries are thought to have cultivated orange trees in Arizona in the early 18th century, while Franciscan missionaries brought the fruit to California in the latter half of that century.

The orange has acquired a vast variety of uses throughout the fruit's long history. Orange pulp contains high levels of vitamin C, offering a daily value of 64% in a single 100 gram serving. Even the rind and the white part of the rind are good sources of vitamin C, with nearly the same amount as the inner flesh. The high vitamin C content in oranges means they do not easily spoil. This is why Dutch, Spanish, and Portuguese seamen cultivated the trees during the Age of Discovery along the trade routes, in order that the fruit's vitamin C would help protect against scurvy.

The orange rind or its juices are used to enhance or garnish recipes. Orange zest – the grated rind – is particularly popular in cooking and baking, due to the zest's strong flavor content.

Of course, oranges are often used in fruit juice for the same reason. Brazil is the world's largest producer of commercial orange juice, but it can also be made at home with a juicer. The high acidity keeps the juice from spoiling too quickly, as well. Moreover, fresh juice is made into the popular frozen orange juice concentrate.

The essential oil is actually a by-product of the juice-making industry. The oil is processed when the peel is cold-pressed and is often used as a flavorant for the food and drink industry. It's also used in the perfume industry, in detergents, household cleaners, hand cleansers, and much more. The fresh aroma provides a sense of cleanliness, while the resulting product is more eco-friendly, substituting synthetic chemicals for natural ones.

The fruit is not the only part of the tree that holds value. Orange blossoms are pleasantly fragrant and tradition deems them a symbol of good fortune, which is why they are often used in weddings, as bouquets or wreaths. In Spain, the blossoms are also used to make tea, while in France or Middle Eastern countries, they are commonly used in cuisine, particularly when it comes to baked goods or desserts. As you can see, the orange has many benefits and uses, and the fruit's essential oil, even more so.

Chemical Components

In order to generate the essential oil from wild orange, the rind must be cold pressed. This results in the oil's key chemical components, which are primarily limonene, alpha pinene, linalool, citronellal, neral, geranial, myrcene, and sabinene.

Main Properties of Wild Orange Essential Oil

Along with the properties previously mentioned in the introduction, wild orange essential oil possesses antioxidant, antibacterial, antifungal, anti-inflammatory, anticancer, antidepressant, antiseptic, antispasmodic, carminative, digestive, sedative, tonic, choleretic, hypotensive, stimulant properties. With such a versatile range, wild orange is well equipped to fight off any pathogen in the body's path.

Wild orange, as mentioned, is composed of limonene, alpha pinene, linalool, citronellal, neral, geranial, myrcene, and sabinene. These components are what instill the enormously beneficial properties within wild orange essential oil. We'll outline these properties below.

Antioxidant

Anything high in antioxidants – whether fruit, beans, or essential oils – is a powerful advocate for your body. Antioxidants both protect against free radicals and repair their damage. What are free radicals? Free radicals are destructive chemicals that invade your body, produced by substances both inside and out. Some free radicals (or oxidants) form through normal bodily reactions, like inflammation, metabolism and aerobic respiration. Other free radicals form outside the body, but enter it due to exposure. These include harmful pollutants, toxins, smoking, alcohol, X-rays, and UV rays, to name a few.

Although our bodies produce their own antioxidants, these often become damaged as we grow older; thus, introducing antioxidants into our bodies allows these nutrients and enzymes to assist in chemical reactions which destroy the oxidants or free radicals. Wild orange essential oil is a moderate antioxidant, aiming to detox the body of free radicals that lead to disease.

Antibacterial

Wild orange's antibacterial properties make it a powerful protectant against diseases produced by bacteria, such as oral, digestive and urinary tract bacterial infection. What's great is that, unlike some prescription drugs, wild orange has no ill effects on bodily health or on the healthy natural flora that exists within the stomach and intestines. Click here, here, and here to read three studies that demonstrate wild orange's antibacterial activity.

Antifungal

While bacteria and viruses are plenty evil, fungi commonly lead to the most deadly infections, whether external or internal. Your ears, throat and nose are the most likely to become infected by fungi, the infections of which can be both excruciating and unsightly. If left untreated, fungal infections can kill, as they may spread to the brain. Wild orange essential oil protects against these infections and more and is particularly effective against skin infections.

Anti-inflammatory

External or internal inflammation can be reduced through the use of wild orange essential oil. For instance, if you or your patient has swollen fingers from arthritis or a swollen knee from a sport's injury, oral application of wild orange essential oil may decrease irritation or redness, while also soothing the pain that accompanies inflammation.

Anticarcinogenic

Wild orange essential oil has been shown to act as an anticarcinogen. An anticarcinogen counters those carcinogens which can potentially produce cancer. Whereas anticarcinomas are used to treat cancer cells after cancer has developed, anticarcinogenics are natural defenses against the development of cancer. Click here to read a study demonstrating wild orange's effects on colon cancer.

Antidepressant

When it comes to psychological issues, the uplifting scent of wild orange essential oil combats negative thoughts and, thereby, depression. The scent is an emotional balancer and can support psychological health. Click here to read a study examining wild orange's effects on psychological health.

Antiseptic

The antiseptic properties of wild orange essential oil

can be reaped topically, applied directly to wounds, or even through burning; the smoke from the oil may help destroy airborne germs. Internal use will help keep the wounds from becoming infections, while external use will support the body's natural function in inhibiting tetanus.

Antispasmodic

The antispasmodic properties of wild orange essential oil make it beneficial to such surgical processes as colonoscopy, gastroscopy, and intraluminally-applied double-contrast barium enema.

Carminative

By supporting the reduction of excess gas buildup and/or removal of gas from the intestines, wild orange essential oil provides relief from abdominal pain, excess sweating, and uncomfortable indigestion.

Digestive

Wild orange boosts the production of absorptive enzymes, the digestibility of nutrients, and the secretion of digestive juices, which aids the digestive tract. Supporting digestion can significantly impact your overall health by increasing those nutrients you absorb from food.

Sedative

As a sedative, wild orange essential oil sedates and

calms by reducing anxiety, excitement or irritability. Though sedatives, alone, do not alleviate pain, they do calm the patient, making them less stressed and more compliant.

Tonic

Wild orange essential oil benefits each of the body's systems, whether nervous, digestive, respiratory or excretory, making it an unbeatable general tonic. The oil also supports the immune system by helping the body absorb nutrients.

Choleretic

A choleretic is a substance that boosts the liver's bile secretion, as well as the volume of solids secreted. In this way, wild orange essential oil further supports good digestive health.

Hypotensive

By relaxing the veins and arteries, wild orange essential oil effectively reduces blood pressure. This boosts circulation and oxygenation to the organ systems and muscles, improving their function. This also supports the metabolism, while further reducing the body's vulnerability to such risks as stroke, heart attack, brain hemorrhaging, or atherosclerosis.

Stimulant

Stimulants are often referred to as "uppers." This is because they produce mental or physical improvements or temporary enhancements of your bodily functions. For instance, you may grow more alert and awake or quicker on your feet after using a stimulant. Wild orange essential oil can provide this temporary boost in mental and physical function, especially when it comes to the immune system.

Common Medicinal Uses

Traditionally used to enhance the body's defenses against infections and diseases, wild orange essential oil remains a significant immune system stimulant, protecting against a number of conditions, whether fungal,or bacterial. Wild orange supports overall health and organ function, while strengthening psychological health. Let's take a closer look at the common uses for this oil.

Immune System Booster

Wild orange is a superb immune system support which boosts circulation and increases white blood cell count. The oil's chemical components deliver incredible antifungal, antibacterial, and stimulant properties, making it akin to an immune shield braced to fight off angry bacterial strains, like MRSA (see study here). With such strong armor, this immune stimulant will ensure that your body is better prepared to protect against deadly infections.

Skin Care

Wild orange oil supports the body's defenses against dermatitis, dryness, and other skin issues. The oil's properties invigorate dull skin, while cleansing and eliminating excess oil. Whether using wild orange essential oil to defy skin aging or to reduce adolescent skin issues, like pimples and acne, the antiseptic and anti-inflammatory properties are superb counter-agents for skin issues. However, it's important to remember that when using any citrus oil topically, you must stay out of direct sunlight for up to 24 hours, as these oils are photosensitive. Click here to read a study that demonstrates wild orange's acne fighting potential.

Anxiety Disorders

Whether it be physical stress or mental anxiety, wild orange's aroma, in conjunction with its therapeutic properties, enable its use in the support of anxiety and other psychological disorders, including upset nerves, anger, melancholy, and depression. The scent of wild orange can help soothe mental fatigue and refresh cognitive function. The oil also induces restful sleep, which helps fortify overall mental well-being. Click here to read a study demonstrating wild orange's effect on anxiety.

Digestive Issues

As a digestive aid, wild orange essential oil's collective properties stimulate digestive enzyme secretion which serves to support issues like constipation, upset stomach, flatulence, indigestion, heartburn, diarrhea, and stomach cramps. As orange is a great additive to water, smoothies, or baked goods, the digestive properties are coupled with an enrichment of culinary flavoring.

Detoxifying Agent

Wild orange essential oil is an effective detoxifying agent. The oil's components eliminate oxidants that enter the body through such environmental inlets as the foods we eat, the products we use, the air we breathe, the water we wash with, and other like factors. Toxins can cause numerous physiological issues, including heart problems, lung or kidney diseases, or even cancer. What wild orange does to eliminate free radicals is to draw the toxins out and transfer them into the urinary tract, where they can be safely removed from the body. Thus, through the oil's high antioxidant content and its ability to stimulate urination, wild orange helps cleanse and detoxify the body's systems.

Muscular and Nervous Spasms

The antispasmodic properties of wild orange essential oil make it useful when it comes to smooth muscle contraction in the gastrointestinal tract or to support the body's defenses against stomach or urinary bladder spasms. Antispasmodics can also support muscular conditions or sports injuries, including acute neck or back pain.

Safety Precautions & Common Applications

Safety

Certain adverse effects may evolve when using pure essential oils. Some essential oils should not be used when pregnant, for example, as they may cause miscarriage. Allergic reactions, too, may occur, especially when applied topically. Always administer an allergy test before committing fully to topical application. When used with other medications, essential oils may react negatively. If you are on any current prescription medications or have a chronic illness, such as high blood pressure, epilepsy or liver disease, then researching the effects of essential oils against your own personal medical history will eliminate any potentially problematic issues.

Wild orange has been approved by the FDA for internal consumption and so can be used as a dietary supplement. If pregnant or breastfeeding, always consult with your physician when using essential oils. Wild orange is also photosensitive, so if used topically, avoid direct sunlight for up to 24 hours. If you have sensitive skin, dilute heavily. If you have sensitive skin, dilute heavily and test before extensive use. Otherwise, dilute 1:1 with a carrier oil. You can apply topically, diffuse or use as a dietary supplement.

Blends

Oftentimes, essential oils are manufactured as blends of several pure oils. For instance, the Protective Blend of certain brands is a mix of cinnamon, clove, rosemary, and eucalyptus. This blend can be used to boost the immune system to help support colds, viruses and flus. The downside to blends is that the more oils added to the mix, the higher the probability your patient may react negatively to the blend if he/she is prone to allergies. There is also the possibility of phototoxicity when working with blends, particularly if they include citrus oils. Be sure to read your labels before administering.

Regardless of these possible effects, essential oils are a viable option for supporting a number of conditions. Those looking to support or maintain their own personal health, or that of their families', should become educated on the uses of essential oils, their natural remedies and the methods of application. Only then can you begin building your kit of essential oils for survival.

Chapter 2:
Recipes for Wild Orange
Essential Oil

In this chapter, we'll offer various recipes for wild orange essential oil, both for pure wild orange applications and blends. For pure applications, we've provided the appropriate dosage and method of administration to support specific ailments, from addiction to viral infections. When it comes to blends, herbalists and aromatherapists often combine wild orange essential oil with vetiver, clove, cinnamon, frankincense, black pepper, ginger, sandalwood, and other citrus oils. We'll offer some fantastic blending options in the second half of this chapter.

Pure Applications

Anxiety

To relieve anxiety, place one drop of wild orange essential oil into your palm and rub your hands together. Place your hand over your nose and mouth and inhale. You can also diffuse throughout your home to alleviate tension and stress.

Calming

Calm anger, stress or nerves by diffusing wild orange essential oil throughout the home. You can also inhale directly or dilute the oil in a 1:1 ratio and apply topically in a full-body massage.

Courage

To enhance confidence and courage, place a drop of wild orange essential oil into your hands, rub your palms together, cup them over your nose, and breathe deeply in and out for several minutes. You can also dilute the oil in a 1:1 ratio and apply topically over the lower abdomen and solar plexus. Use daily for the best results.

Constipation

To help relieve constipation, dilute wild orange essential oil in a 1:1 ratio with a carrier oil and massage in a clockwise motion over the abdomen twice daily.

Cooking

You can use wild orange essential oil in cooking, as it's generally regarded as safe by the FDA. Orange is a nice addition to frostings, smoothies, or baking. One drop (or less) to begin with; add more to taste. A little oil goes a long way.

Diarrhea

If you're experiencing diarrhea, wild orange essential oil is the answer. Apply topically by diluting the oil in a 1:1 ratio with a carrier oil and massaging it into the abdomen in a counterclockwise motion twice daily, or place a drop of the oil in your drinking water throughout the day.

Digestive Aid

Wild orange essential oil aids the digestive tract and can be taken orally or topically. Place a drop into your drinking water for internal administration or dilute the oil in a 1:1 ratio with a carrier oil and apply topically to the abdomen and into the reflex points of the feet. You can also diffuse throughout the home for added support.

Emotional Balance

Wild orange essential oil can help provide emotional balance. Dilute 1 drop of the oil in 1 tablespoon of a carrier oil and apply topically, massaging the combo into the chest.

You can also administer the oil aromatically by diffusing or inhaling directly from the bottle.

Fear

To help eliminate unwarranted fear, dilute wild orange essential oil in a 1:1 ratio with a carrier oil and apply topically, massaging over the solar plexus and the heart. You can also administer aromatically, diffusing throughout the home or inhaling directly from the bottle.

Heartburn

Relieve heartburn by diluting wild orange essential oil in a 1:1 ratio with a carrier oil and massaging it in a downward motion from throat to stomach, as well as across the arches and soles of the feet. You can also add a drop to your drinking water and take orally.

Heart Palpitations

To protect against heart palpitations, dilute wild orange essential oil in a 1:1 ratio with a carrier oil and apply topically, massaging over the heart and into the reflex points of the feet up to three times a day. For added support, diffuse throughout the room.

Immune Stimulant

Give your immune system a leg up by regularly diffusing wild orange essential oil throughout your home, especially during cold and flu season. The scent also uplifts and boosts energy. Alternatively, you can add a couple drops to your bathwater or dilute in a 1:1 ratio with a carrier oil and apply topically, massaging the oil into the feet. If you'd prefer the steam method, steam two drops of wild orange essential oil in a pan of water, remove the steaming pan from the stove, pour into a bowl, place a towel over your head and inhale. If you don't feel it's done its job the first time, you can reheat that same water and use it once more without adding more oil.

Insomnia

Although wild orange can often be stimulating, the scent can also calm and relax, helping to relieve insomnia. In order to trigger nervous system response, dilute in a 1:1 ratio with a carrier oil and apply topically to the reflex points in the feet. You might also diffuse or place a couple drops on your pillow or sheets.

Jaundice

For those suffering from jaundice, support the issue with a topical blend. Dilute 1 drop of wild orange essential oil with 1 teaspoon of a carrier oil and massage into the reflex points of the feet and over the full body.

Menopause

Support the body's natural defenses against menopausal symptoms by diluting wild orange essential oil in a 1:1 ratio with a carrier oil and applying topically over the chest, lower abdomen, base and front of the neck, and into the soles of the feet. You can also diffuse throughout the home to maintain hormonal balance.

Mouth Ulcers

Support the body's natural defenses against mouth ulcers by placing a drop of wild orange essential oil in a glass of water and rinsing the mouth three times daily.

Nervousness

Nervousness can be calmed through diffusing or directly inhaling wild orange essential oil. You can also pour a drop into your hands, rub your palms together, cup them over your nose, and breathe deeply in and out for several minutes. For topical administration, dilute the oil in a 1:1 ratio with a carrier oil and massage over the abdomen.

Skin (Dry, Sensitive, Eczema, Dermatitis, etc)

Wild orange essential oil can support all types of skin conditions. Dilute wild orange essential oil in a 1:1 ratio with a carrier oil and apply topically to the affected area. You can also add a drop of wild orange to your daily skin regimen.

Uplifting

Like most citrus scents, wild orange essential oil is naturally uplifting. To absorb the oil's mood balancing effects, diffuse regularly throughout the home or, for quick pick-me-ups, pour a drop into your hands, rub your palms together, cup them over your nose, and breathe deeply in and out for several minutes.

Withdrawal

If you're feeling a sense of withdrawal, stimulate confidence, safety, and security by pouring a drop into your hands, rubbing your palms together, cupping them over your nose, and breathing deeply in and out for several minutes. For topical administration, dilute the oil in a 1:1 ratio with a carrier oil and massage into the reflex points of the feet.

Blends

Aphrodisiac Massage Blend

Ingredients

- 2 drops Black Pepper Essential Oil

- 2 drops Ginger Essential Oil

- 3 drops Wild Orange Essential Oil

- 3 drops Rosemary Essential Oil

- 4 drops Ylang Ylang Essential Oil

- 4 drops Bergamot Essential Oil

- 4 drops Sandalwood Essential Oil

- 4 ounces Carrier Oil (fractionated coconut oil recommended)

Directions

To stimulate sexual arousal for men and women, combine all ingredients in a small bowl, blending well. Apply in a full body massage or into the reflex points. Store in a glass bottle.

Aphrodisiac Scent

Ingredients

- 1 drop Clove Essential Oil

- 1 drop Cassia Essential Oil

- 3 drops Wild Orange Essential Oil

- 1 tsp Carrier Oil

Directions

In a small bowl or container, mix all ingredients until well combined. Apply to the pulse points for an attractive scent.

Bedside Pillow Spray

Ingredients

- 1 drop Chamomile Essential Oil

- 1 drop Wild Orange Essential Oil

- 1 drop Ylang Ylang Essential Oil

- 2 drops Lavender Essential Oil

- 15 mL Distilled Water

Directions

To ease yourself or your family members into a dreamless sleep, combine all ingredients in spray bottle and shake well. Spritz over pillow cases and let dry before bed time.

Calming Bath Blend

Ingredients

- 1 drop Patchouli Essential Oil

- 2 drops Wild Orange Essential Oil

- 3 drops Lavender Essential Oil

Directions

To calm nerves and unwind after a long day, add all
ingredients to your bathwater and stir to disperse.
Then inhale deeply while you soak for 20 minutes, but
avoid getting water in your eyes, as it may sting.

Calming Massage

Ingredients

- 4 drops Neroli Essential Oil

- 5 drops Wild Orange Essential Oil

- 6 drops Petitgrain Essential Oil

- 15 mL Carrier Oil

Directions

To calm nerves or stress, combine all ingredients in a small bowl or glass jar and mix well. Apply in a full-body massage.

Cheery Citrus Diffusion Blend

Ingredients

- 1 drop Wild Orange Essential Oil

- 1 drop Tangerine Essential Oil

- 1 drop Lime Essential Oil

- 2 drops Lemon Essential Oil

- 3 drops Grapefruit Essential Oil

Directions

For a fresh, uplifting, cheerful scent, combine all ingredients in your diffuser and use as normal.

Cheery Citrus Spray

Ingredients

- 1 drop Nutmeg Essential Oil

- 1 drop Clary Sage Essential Oil

- 2 drops Lavender Essential Oil

- 3 drops Lemon Essential Oil

- 3 drops Orange Essential Oil

- 3 drops Lime Essential Oil

- 2 ounces Witch Hazel

Directions

For a cheerful citrus scent that uplifts the mood, combine all ingredients in a dark colored glass spray bottle, shake well, and use as normal. The combination can also be applied to furniture dusting. Shake well before each use.

Cheery Diffusion Blend

Ingredients

- 4 drops Wild Orange Essential Oil

- 4 drops Frankincense Essential Oil

- 2 drops Clove Bud Essential Oil

Directions

For a warm, cheerful scent, combine all ingredients in your diffuser and use as normal. Great choice to lift winter or seasonal spirits.

Chills & Colds Warming Bath Blend

Ingredients

- 2 drops Ginger Essential Oil

- 2 drops Benzoin Essential Oil

- 2 drops Wild Orange Essential Oil

- 1 Tbsp Grapeseed Oil

Directions

For a bath that warms you to the bones, add all ingredients to your bathwater and stir to disperse. Then inhale deeply while you soak for 20 minutes, but avoid getting water in your eyes, as it may sting. Great during cold season.

Circulation Stimulant

Ingredients

4 drops Cypress Essential Oil

2 drops Rosemary Essential Oil

2 drops Cilantro Essential Oil

2 drops Wild Orange Essential Oil

½ ounce Coconut Oil

Directions

To stimulate circulation, combine all ingredients in a small container, mixing until well blended. Apply topically to the ankles towards the heart.

De-stress Massage

Ingredients

- 5 drops Geranium Essential Oil
- 5 drops Coriander Essential Oil
- 5 drops Lavender Essential Oil
- 3 drops Wild Orange Essential Oil
- 2 ounces Sweet Almond Oil

Directions

To wind down, de-stress, and combat anxiety, combine all ingredients in a small bowl or glass jar and mix well. Apply in a full-body massage.

Energy Booster

Ingredients

- 10 drops Orange Essential Oil

- 10 drops Cinnamon Essential Oil

- 10 drops Black Pepper Essential Oil

Directions

Diffuse blend throughout your home to stimulate energy.

Flea & Tick Repellant

Ingredients

- 1 drop Thyme Essential Oil

- 1 drop Cedarwood Essential Oil

- 3 drops Citronella Essential Oil

- 3 drops Lavender Essential Oil

- 4 drops Wild Orange Essential Oil

- ½ tsp Alcohol

Directions

To relieve your pets of fleas and ticks, place all ingredients into a small bowl or container and blend thoroughly. Apply topically, massaging into the affected area.

Harmonious Diffusion Blend

Ingredients

- 1 drops Grapefruit Essential Oil

- 1 drop Ylang Ylang Essential Oil

- 1 drop Wild Orange Essential Oil

- 2 drops Patchouli Essential Oil

- 3 drops Bergamot Essential Oil

Directions

To support harmony in a tense home or mind, combine all ingredients in your diffuser and use as normal.

Jetlag Fix

Ingredients

- 10 drops Wild Orange Essential Oil

- 10 drops Spruce Essential Oil

- 5 drops Lavender Essential Oil

- 1 ounce Jojoba Oil

Directions

To combat jetlag, combine all ingredients in a small bowl or container, blending well. Apply topically in a full-body massage and into the reflex points of the feet.

Joyful Mist

Ingredients

- 10 drops Frankincense Essential Oil

- 8 drops Orange Essential Oil

- 7 drops Clary Sage Essential Oil

- 48 mL Distilled Water

- 1 mL Vodka

Directions

For a joyful mist spray, combine ingredients in a 50mL glass spray bottle and spray throughout your room, study, or vehicle at the end of a tough day. Shake well before each use.

Libido Diffusion Blend

Ingredients

- 3-4 drops Ylang Ylang Essential Oil

- 1 drop Wild Orange Essential Oil

Directions

To stimulate libido, add all ingredients to a diffuser and inhale the aromatic scent. You can also combine this duo with a carrier oil and apply topically, massaging over the wrists and thyroid, as well as behind the ears.

Pick-me-up Diffusion Blend

Ingredients

- 3 drops Cinnamon Essential Oil

- 3 drops Ylang Ylang Essential Oil

- 5 drops Patchouli Essential Oil

- 8 drops Wild Orange Essential Oil

- 3.5 ounces Carrier Oil

Directions

For a romantic and relaxing scent, combine all ingredients in a small bowl or container, blending well. To use as a perfume, apply to the pulse points or administer in a full-body massage.

Stress Relief

Ingredients

- 25 drops Wild Orange Essential Oil

- 20 drops Grapefruit Essential Oil

- 15 drops Frankincense Essential Oil

- 15 drops Bergamot Essential Oil

- 10 drops Clary Sage Essential Oil

- 10 drops Lemon Essential Oil

Directions

To help focus concentration, diffuse throughout the home or office.

Uplifting Scent

Ingredients

3 drops Clary Sage Essential Oil

3 drops Wild Orange Essential Oil

2 drops Ylang Ylang Essential Oil

Directions

For a smooth, uplifting scent to support emotional and mental health, combine all ingredients in your diffuser and use as normal.

Chapter 3:
Wild Orange Essential Oil Studies

Many studies have been done on essential oils to uncover and prove their therapeutic qualities. In the case of the great number of wild orange studies, many of the properties attributed to the essential oil (noted in this book and elsewhere) are quite often validated through the research from accredited universities and published by reputable scientific journals. In this chapter, we'll discuss a small portion of these studies. It's important to note that our knowledge of essential oils is constantly evolving. Keep up with any recent research, as it may turn up even further valuable uses for these miracle oils.

Study 1 – Acne

In this study published by Biomedica, the effects of wild orange essential oil on acne were examined, with the following results: "Currently, the antimicrobial resistance has developed in bacterial strains involved in the development of acne. Therefore, alternatives to antibiotic treatment have become necessary...Gel formulations were designed based on essential oils and acetic acid, and their effectiveness was evaluated in patients affected by acne...The results were ranked good to excellent, particularly for the acetic acid mixture, which achieved improvements of 75%. This appeared to be a result of their joint antiseptic and keratolytic activity."

This study sought an alternative to antibiotic acne treatments, as certain acne bacterial strains are now showing antimicrobial resistance to current solutions. The study formed three gel formulas to test on four groups with seven patients each, 28 volunteers total. The gel formulas included antibacterial essential oils (basil and wild orange), a keratolytic medication, the essential oils combined with acetic acid, and the keratolytic medication combined with acetic acid. The volunteers were evaluated weekly and, although the acne condition improved in all groups (with anywhere from 43-75% lesion clearance), those groups using essential oil formulas enjoyed chemically and physically stable results. The study demonstrates wild orange essential oil's antibacterial acne-fighting potential.

Reference:

http://www.ncbi.nlm.nih.gov/pubmed/23235794]

http://www.scielo.org.co/scielo.php?script=sci_pdf&pid=
S0120-41572012000100014&lng=en&nrm=iso&tlng=es]

Study 2 – Antimicrobial Activity

In this study published by Evidence-Based Complementary and Alternative Medicine, the synergistic effects of wild orange essential oil in combination with lavender were examined, with the following results: "The antimicrobial activity of Lavandula angustifolia essential oil was assessed in combination with 45 other oils to establish possible interactive properties…the most favorable interactions were when L. angustifolia was combined with Cinnamomum zeylanicum or with Citrus sinensis, against C. albicans and S. aureus, respectively…Within the field of aromatherapy, essential oils are commonly employed in mixtures for the treatment of infectious diseases; however, very little evidence exists to support the use in combination. This study lends some credence to the concomitant use of essential oils blended with lavender."

The objective of this study was to demonstrate the synergistic effect of two oils combined, in this case lavender and wild orange. Out of 45 combinations, the study found that in 1:1 ratios, the synergistic antibacterial effect of the lavender-orange oil combo against Staphylococcus aureus was the most favorable. S. aureus is Gram-positive bacterium. Although S. aureus is part of the normal human skin flora and respiratory tract and is not typically pathogenic, those with compromised immune systems can potentially develop an infection from the bacteria. When it becomes pathogenic, S. aureus produces respiratory issues like sinusitis, skin infections, and even food poisoning. This study demonstrates the efficacy of a lavender-orange essential oil blend against this strain of bacteria.

Reference
http://www.ncbi.nlm.nih.gov/pubmed/23737850]

http://www.ncbi.nlm.nih.gov/pmc/articles/PMC3666441/pdf/ECAM2013-852049.pdf]

Study 3 – Anxiety Disorders

In this study published by PLOS One, the anxiolytic effects of wild orange essential oil were examined, with the following results: "Anxiety disorders are the most prevalent psychiatric disorders and affect a great number of people worldwide. Essential oils, take effects through inhalation or topical application, are believed to enhance physical, emotional, and spiritual well-being. Although clinical studies suggest that the use of essential oils may have therapeutic potential, evidence for the efficacy of essential oils in treating medical conditions remains poor, with a particular lack of studies employing rigorous analytical methods that capture its identifiable impact on human biology…This study demonstrates, for the first time, that the metabonomics approach can capture the subtle metabolic changes resulting from exposure to essential oils and provide the basis for pinpointing affected pathways in anxiety-related behavior, which will lead to an improved mechanistic understanding of anxiolytic effect of essential oils."

The study examined the anxiolytic effects of four aromatic plants – lavandula angustifolia, salvia sclarea, santalum album, and citrus sinensis – in order to better understand how essential oils biologically affect anxiety. The metabolic changes of the rats tested were found in the brain tissue and urinary metabolites. After inducing anxiety via an elevated plus maze, the metabolic level alterations in the brain included reduced neurotransmitter levels, fatty acids, amino acids, and increased carbohydrates. In the urine, there were also elevated levels of carbohydrates, aspartate, nucleosides, and organic acids. After ten days of aromatherapy, these metabolic levels were reduced significantly. This indicates that essential oil aromatherapy has a distinct biological effect, essentially returning metabolic levels back to pre-anxiety levels.

Reference
http://www.ncbi.nlm.nih.gov/pubmed/22984571]

http://www.ncbi.nlm.nih.gov/pmc/articles/PMC3440318/pdf/pone.0044830.pdf

Study 4 – Colon Cancer

In this study published in Life Science, the anticancer properties of wild orange essential oil were examined, with the following results: "To identify the chemical constituents of volatile oil from blood orange (Citrus sinensis (L) Osbeck) and understand the possible mechanisms of inhibition of colon cancer cell proliferation…The results of this study provide persuasive evidence of the apoptotic and anti-angiogenesis potential of BVOE in colon cancer cells. The extent of induction of apoptosis and inhibition of angiogenesis suggest that BVOE may offer great potential for prevention of cancer and may be appropriate for further studies."

This study endeavored to determine the viability of wild orange essential oil in inhibiting colon cancer cells. In the study, an emulsion of the essential oil was created and tested on colon cancer cells and was found to induce apoptosis in these cells. In multicellular organisms, apoptosis is the process of programmed cell death. In the case of cancer, an insufficient amount of apoptosis results in an unmanageable growth of cancer cells, thus the cell death induced by wild orange essential oil may be applicable to controlling the cancer's growth. Moreover, wild orange essential oil also demonstrated antiangiogenic activity. Although angiogenesis is normal and crucial when it comes to wound healing, growth, and development, it is also partially responsible for transitioning benign tumors into malignant ones. This is why cancer patients are treated with angiogenesis inhibitors. Wild orange essential oil was shown to be a natural antiangiogenic, helping to protect against the benign to malignant transition. Overall, the study demonstrates the efficacy of using wild orange to help fortify the body's defenses against colon cancer.

Reference
http://www.ncbi.nlm.nih.gov/pubmed/22935404]

Study 5 – Antibacterial Activity

In this study published in BMC Complementary & Alternative Medicine , the antibacterial effects of wild orange essential oil were examined, with the following results: "Staphylococcus aureus is the pathogen most often and prevalently involved in skin and soft tissue infections. In recent decades outbreaks of methicillin-resistant S. aureus (MRSA) have created major problems for skin therapy, and burn and wound care units. Topical antimicrobials are most important component of wound infection therapy. Alternative therapies are being sought for treatment of MRSA and one area of interest is the use of essential oils. With the increasing interest in the use and application of natural products, we screened the potential application of terpeneless cold pressed Valencia orange oil (CPV) for topical therapy against MRSA using an in vitro dressing model and skin keratinocyte cell culture model…At lower concentration addition of CPV to keratinocytes infected with MRSA and VISA rapidly killed the bacterial cells without causing any toxic effect to the keratinocytes. Therefore, the results of this study warrant further in vivo study to evaluate the potential of CPV as a topical antistaphylococcal agent."

As mentioned in the first study, S. aureus is Gram-positive bacterium. Methicillin-resistant Staphylococcus aureus (MRSA) is any strain of S. aureus that's naturally developed a resistance to antibiotics, including penicillin. This hospital-acquired infection is now limitedly endemic.

Being resistant to standard medications, these strains –
although not more virulent than other S. aureus strains –
may result in infections that are tough to treat. Hospitals,
nursing homes, and prisons largely house MRSA, and
patients with weak immune systems and open wounds are
most at risk.

The study found that wild orange essential oil had an
inhibitory effect on MRSA strains, without any cytotoxic
effect on skin cells. These results indicate that wild orange
essential oil could potentially be used as an antibacterial
agent for this strain of bacteria.

Reference
http://www.ncbi.nlm.nih.gov/pubmed/22894560]

http://www.ncbi.nlm.nih.gov/pmc/articles/PMC3522527/
pdf/1472-6882-12-125.pdf]

Study 6 – Insecticidal Activity

In this study available on PubMed, the insecticidal activity of wild orange essential oil was examined, with the following results: "Insecticidal activity of the essential oils (EOs) isolated from…Citrus sinensis…aromatic plants, grown in Colombia (Bucaramanga, Santander)…were evaluated on Aedes (Stegomyia) aegypti Rockefeller larvae…The following values were obtained for C. flexuosus (LC50 = 17.1 ppm); C. sinensis (LC50 = 20.6 ppm)…The EO from C. flexuosus, with citral (geranial + neral) as main component, showed the highest larvicidal activity."

Prevalent primarily in the tropics, dengue fever affects between 50 and 528 million people annually and is endemic in over 110 countries. The infection is transmitted via mosquitoes which carry the dengue virus, among them the Ae. aegypti species. The resulting symptoms of the viral disease include joint and muscle pain, fever, and skin rash which is akin to the measles. The disease can sometimes escalate into dengue hemorrhagic fever or dengue shock syndrome, each far more fatal than common dengue fever. There is no commercial vaccine for dengue fever, therefore eliminating the mosquitoes' habitats and reducing exposure to bites is the primary preventative measure. Treatment of dengue fever, as well, is supported primarily through rehydration with no pharmaceutical medication yet developed to target the virus directly (although medications are in development).

According to this study, wild orange essential oil shows promise in the preventative department. The oil demonstrated superior repellent properties against the larvae of Ae. aegypti, the mosquito species that commonly carries the virus, making it an effective potential mosquito control in areas where dengue fever is endemic.

Reference & Photo Credit:
http://www.ncbi.nlm.nih.gov/pubmed/24781026]

Chapter 4:
The Ins & Outs of Essential Oils

Where do essential oils come from?

Plants and plant species naturally produce essential oils for various reasons, one being to draw pollinator insects to them, another being to repel invading organisms (bacteria, animals). A number of chemical compounds compose each plant's essential oil, and the combination of these compounds is specific to each oil, which then instills in the oil its own unique properties. Essential oils can be harnessed from all sorts of plant components, including flowers, leaves, bark, fruit, roots, and resin. For instance, cinnamon oil is harnessed from bark, lemon oil from the peel, and lavender oil from lavender flowers. Certain plants can produce a few chemical variants of the same essential oil, which are acquired from different parts of the plant. Some of these parts produce a large amount of oil, while others produce just a smidgen. The oil's quality and potency depends upon a number of factors, including the subspecies of the plant, its soil conditions, the time of year and even the time of day you harvest it.

How are essential oils extracted?

Essential oils can be extracted from plants through various methods, including pressing, distillation, solvent and maceration. Let's take a brief look at each:

Pressing Method

Commonly used with citrus fruit, the pressing method extracts the oil through a technique which involves pushing the fruit peels through a press. Oily fruits and plants are best suited for this technique. Orange oil, for example, is extracted from orange skins through the pressing method.

Distillation Method

This technique harkens back to the days of old-timey moonshiners, as the same sort of method used to create strong liquor can be used to extract essential oils. Using a still, boiled water and plant materials will create steam which is then cooled by coils and condensed into a combination of water and oil. This combination doesn't mix, so the oil can then be extracted from it.

Solvent Method

Through a multi-step process, certain plant and flower oils can be extracted using alcohol and other solvents, which extort the essential oil from the plant materials.

Maceration Method

When a "carrier" or fixed oil or lard is mixed with the plant material and set out in the sun, over a period of time, the carrier oil is infused with the plant's essence. Heat sources, other than the sun, are often used to speed the process. Throughout the process, more plant material is added to produce a more potent oil.

How do you use essential oils?

Although some studies about the effectiveness of essential oils are conducted by small companies or even individuals, a number of them are conducted by the food and cosmetic industries. In general, the pharmaceutical industry shows next to no interest in herbal medicine, primarily because there are few options to patent such products. Being as such, the product's lack of profitability results in a lack of research funding. Regardless, the historical uses of essential oils tell us what we need to know: these oils have been effectively administered for centuries. The therapeutic qualifications of essential oils can be plotted in the survival of the human race across cultures and generations.

Another reason that studies on essential oils have not resulted in much conclusive evidence as to their overall effectiveness is because definitive results are sometimes difficult to prove, as the quality of each batch of oil can vary for a number of reasons. One is that essential oils are impossible to standardize. As mentioned above, even the slightest variance in soil conditions and the time of harvesting – as well as innumerable other factors – will produce a different product quality and potency. In addition, essential oils are often obtained from various species of the same plant; Eucalyptus radiata and Eucalyptus globulus can both be used in the making of therapeutic-grade eucalyptus oil and, as a result, they may have slightly different properties and degrees of strength or effectiveness.

Just as there are a number of methods by which to extract essential oils, there are a number of methods to administer them therapeutically. The variety of chemical compounds in each essential oil means that their benefits and applications also vary across the board. Below are a few of these methods.

Topical Administration

Direct application of many essential oils works like a sponge, as skin sops up chemicals and other things (like sunlight, for instance). Topical application is best when you want to clear up an ailment on the skin's surface or in the underlying muscle tissue. When applying topically, you may either massage the oil into the skin or simply dab on the skin for therapeutic results. You might combine the essential oil with a carrier oil for topical use in order to dilute its potency. This is safer, as the oil is so concentrated. You may support your body's defenses against rash or muscle pain in this manner, but you should always test your patient for allergies before applying. Adverse effects are produced by natural chemicals as much as synthetic ones; poison ivy, for example.

To test for allergens, place a drop or two on your patient's inner forearm. If a rash develops within 12 to 24 hours, then the patient is allergic. In addition, phototoxicity – sun exposure resulting in an exacerbated burn – may be an issue when citrus oils are applied topically. So one must proceed with caution when applying essential oils using this method.

Inhalation Therapy

Commonly known as "aromatherapy", this essential oil application is effective for inner ailments, like sore throat or cold. In a steaming bowl of distilled or sterilized water, add a few drops of essential oil and, with a towel over your head, bend over the bowl and inhale. The towel captures the vapors, making the technique even more effective. Essential oils can also be placed in a diffuser or potpourri throughout a room to produce somewhat diluted therapeutic effects.

Ingestion

When using this method, proceed with caution. Direct ingestion of essential oils must be monitored and applied in small doses that are diluted in a tablespoon or more of any carrier oil – olive oil, for example. If you are unsure of dosage amounts, make a tea with the relevant herb instead. Although the effects of this diluted use may be weaker, this application is a better alternative than an overdose of essential oils.

What are the general benefits of using essential oils?

Replacement for Prescription Drugs

One practical benefit for using essential oils is, of course, their substitutive nature; they can replace Rx drugs, which is the ultimate reason to educate yourself on their administration and to begin stockpiling your essential oil supply. One of the potential threats of economic or social collapse is the lack of resources, and primarily the inability to procure prescription drugs. Being as such, finding suitable supplements should be a priority when preparing for the worst.

Their portability is also a major bonus when it comes to survival prepping. The fact that these ultra-concentrated oils take up little-to-no space makes toting them to your shelter all the simpler should the need arise. And, because essential oils are highly concentrated, the application used in most methods of administration requires only a drop or two of oil, which means that tiny bottle will be long-lasting.

Cost Effective Supplement

Though money may be the last thing on your mind when it comes to prepping for a survival situation (money may even be obsolete in the event of social collapse), it is worth noting that the expense of essential oils pales in comparison to prescription drugs. Essential oils are a cost effective supplement to prescription medicine.

No Expiration Date

Another benefit of essential oils is that they do not expire, neither do they have "proper storage" requirements. A number of medicines and medicinal products must be replaced every couple years, so this sets essential oils ahead of the pack when it comes to shelf life.

Versatility

Essential oils also offer great versatility. Apart from providing therapeutic benefits, essential oils can be repurposed for household and hygienic applications. For instance, if you're looking for something that might serve your dental hygiene needs in a time of crisis, the protective oil blend is your go-to essential oil. If you want to maintain your skin's tone and condition, frankincense and lavender will do the trick; the latter also serves as sunscreen, so you can inhibit sun damage as well.

When it comes to the house or shelter, you can use essential oils to deodorize, which will come in handy in a disaster scenario where things might start to smell fishy due to lack of proper utilities and care. For example, after the 2011 tsunami and the subsequent nuclear reactor meltdown in Japan, a nurse named Risa Nakahira used essential oils to deodorize and sanitize putrid public bathrooms in overpopulated evacuation facilities. As relief workers searched for survivors, often wading through debris and decay, Nakahira also deodorized their boots and masks using essential oils. The possibilities of these natural oils are endless.

They are also versatile when it comes to the range of patients they're capable of supporting. The wellness of everyone from your great grandfather to your infant baby can be fortified with the aid of essential oils in the appropriate dosage. They even come in handy when supporting the wellness of livestock or pets. From teething infants to dementia in the elderly, from teenagers with acne to dogs with urinary tract infections, essential oils can serve any patient with nearly any ailment.

Conclusion

Now that you know all about what wild orange essential oil can do for you – where it originates, how it's extracted, its benefits and properties, and the different methods of administration – you can use it confidently to support the body's defenses against health issues and start to assemble a kit of essential oils for survival. Essential oils can be purchased online or at your local holistic treatment store.

The various benefits of essential oils and their properties are countless. To build your own kit, first focus on acquiring the essential oils which may bear more relevance to your health issues or the potential health threats within your environment. When it comes to cold and flu season, for instance, wild orange essential oil will be one of your more crucial oils, due to its immune-supportive properties.

Used as a supplement or as your go-to for anxiety disorders, skin care, or detoxification, the application of wild orange essential oil in medicine has survived for centuries and will survive centuries more. When it comes down to it, you don't need to rely on pharmaceuticals; essential oils, herbs, and plenty of other natural ingredients can be used to help support any number of health issues, whether ailment or injury.

Essential oils are essential to your survival in the case

of viral outbreak, social collapse or natural disaster because, when the SHTF, your access to pharmaceuticals will likely either be limited or eliminated altogether. Alternatives to our modern-day standard will equate survival when no other option exists. And when it comes to a life-or-death situation, you can't let your health decline, no matter the state of the world.

DISCLAIMER AND/OR LEGAL NOTICES: Every effort has been made to accurately represent this book and it's potential. Results vary with every individual, and your results may or may not be different from those depicted. No promises, guarantees or warranties, whether stated or implied, have been made that you will produce any specific result from this book. Your efforts are individual and unique, and may vary from those shown. Your success depends on your efforts, background and motivation.

The material in this publication is provided for educational and informational purposes only and is not intended as medical advice. The information contained in this book should not be used to diagnose or treat any illness, metabolic disorder, disease or health problem. Always consult your physician or healthcare provider before beginning any nutrition or exercise program. Use of the programs, advice, and information contained in this book is at the sole choice and risk of the reader.